Memories & Milestones

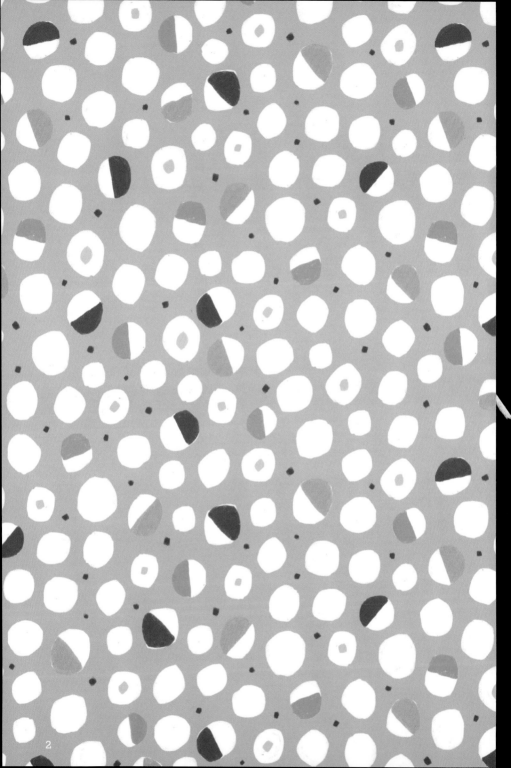

So many beautiful things are ahead.

New wonders and tender wishes. Promises to keep and new dreams to carry. Courage and strength and so much beauty and affection for you to share. An incredible amount of love is just ahead too. Love for a small, sweet life you don't yet know, but can feel in every part of you. Your belly will grow— and with it, your heart. And the most beautiful gift for both of you is that this is just the beginning...

Sometimes the smallest

things take up the

most room in our hearts.

A. A. MILNE

We're Growing!

WEEK:

You're the size of a:

_____
_____
_____
_____
_____
_____
_____
_____
_____
_____
_____

Ways you've grown and developed recently:

_____
_____
_____
_____
_____
_____
_____
_____
_____
_____
_____
_____
_____

Right now, I'm most looking forward to:

I'm getting ready for you by:

NOTES

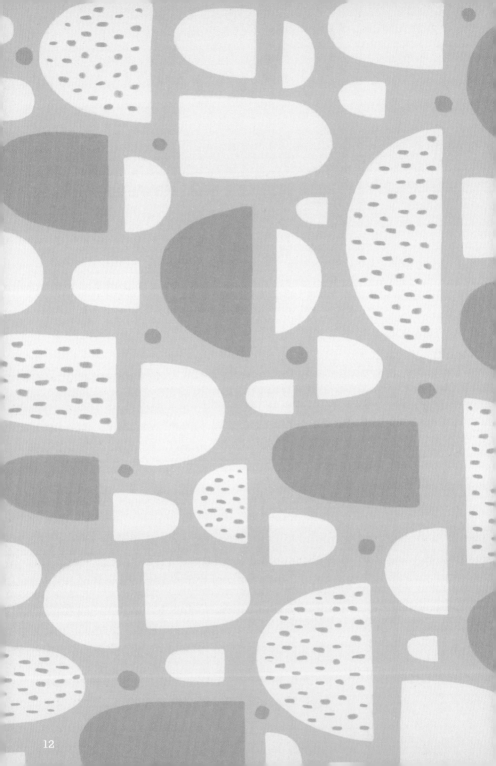

A new baby is like the beginning of all things— wonder, hope, a dream of possibilities.

EDA LESHAN

I have
so many
dreams
for you.

Some of my favorites to think about are...

The day I discovered I was pregnant:

_____

_____

_____

_____

_____

_____

_____

_____

_____

_____

_____

_____

_____

_____

_____

_____

_____

_____

_____

_____

_____

_____

_____

_____

Who I told first:

_____

_____

_____

How I shared the news:

_____
_____
_____
_____
_____
_____
_____
_____
_____
_____
_____
_____
_____
_____
_____
_____
_____
_____
_____
_____

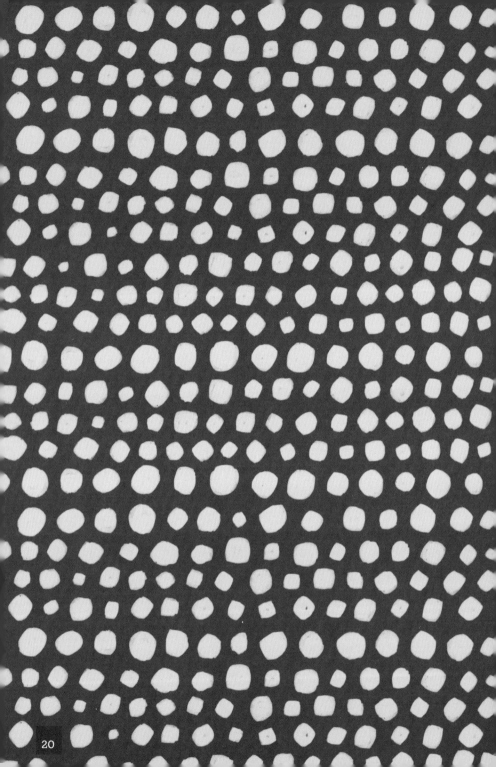

...those things you hear about having a baby and motherhood— all of them are true. And all of them are the most beautiful things you will ever experience.

PENÉLOPE CRUZ

We're Growing!

WEEK:

You're the size of a:

These days I'm feeling:

Ways you've grown and developed recently:

Right now, I'm most looking forward to:

I'm getting ready for you by:

NOTES

& THINGS TO REMEMBER

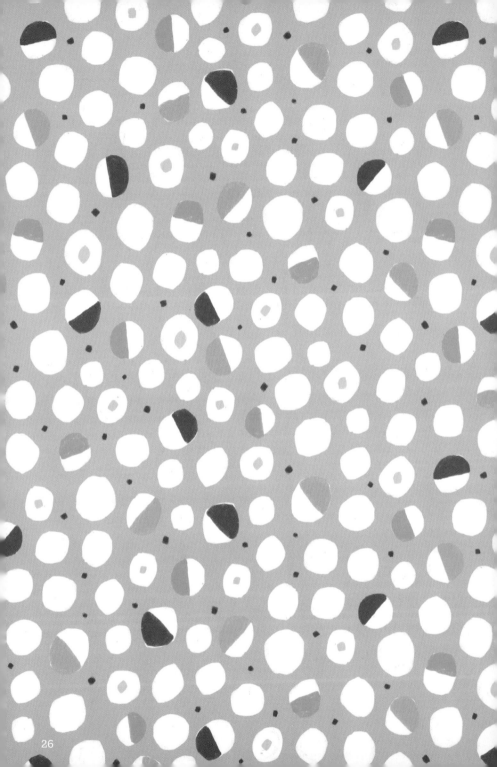

There is such a special sweetness in being able to participate in creation.

PAMELA S. NADAV

There are lots of
people helping me
prepare for you...

Friends, family, and caregivers, including:

Making the decision
to have a child, it's
momentous. It is to decide
forever to have your
heart go walking around
outside your body.

ELIZABETH STONE

Many experiences have happened in my life to prepare me for having you. Some of them are...

_____
_____
_____
_____
_____
_____
_____
_____
_____
_____
_____
_____
_____
_____
_____
_____
_____
_____
_____
_____
_____
_____

There is a miracle in
every new beginning.

HERMANN HESSE

We're Growing!

WEEK:

You're the size of a:

These days I'm feeling:

Ways you've grown and developed recently:

Right now, I'm most looking forward to:

I'm getting ready for you by:

NOTES

I want so many things!

These are some of my cravings:

Our friends and family think we're having a:

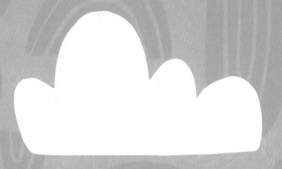

I think you're going to be a:

Because:

The life of a mother
is the life of a child:
you are two blossoms
on a single branch.

KAREN MAEZEN MILLER

We're Growing!

WEEK:

You're the size of a:

These days I'm feeling:

_____

_____

_____

_____

_____

_____

_____

_____

_____

_____

_____

Ways you've grown and developed recently:

_____

_____

_____

_____

_____

_____

_____

_____

_____

_____

_____

_____

_____

Right now, I'm most looking forward to:

I'm getting ready for you by:

NOTES

& THINGS TO REMEMBER

Nicknames for you:

A mother's joy begins when
new life is stirring inside,
when a tiny heartbeat is heard
for the very first time, and a
playful kick reminds her
that she is never alone.

UNKNOWN

I heard your heartbeat
for the first time on...

___ / ___ / ___

It sounded like...

Go to work?

Stay at home?

After you're born, my hope is to...

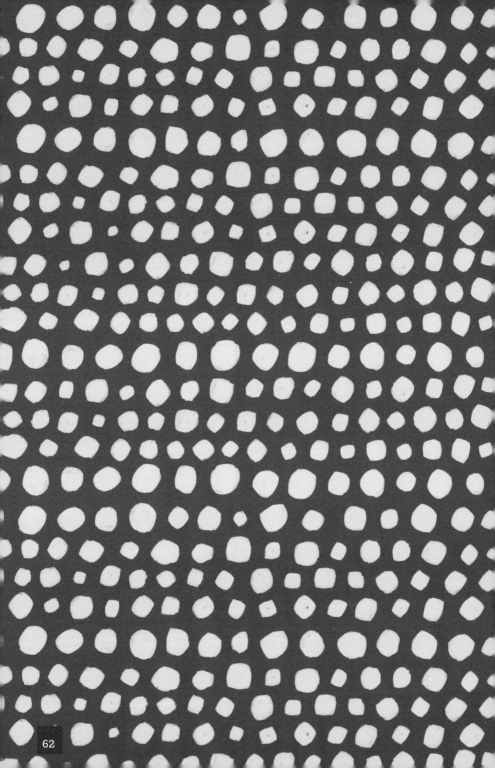

To be pregnant is to be
vitally alive... a time
of transition, growth, and
profound beginnings.

ANNE CHRISTIAN BUCHANAN
& DEBRA K. KINGSPORN

We're Growing!

WEEK:

You're the size of a:

These days I'm feeling:

_____

_____

_____

_____

_____

_____

_____

_____

_____

_____

Ways you've grown and developed recently:

_____

_____

_____

_____

_____

_____

_____

_____

_____

_____

_____

Right now, I'm most looking forward to:

I'm getting ready for you by:

NOTES

& THINGS TO REMEMBER

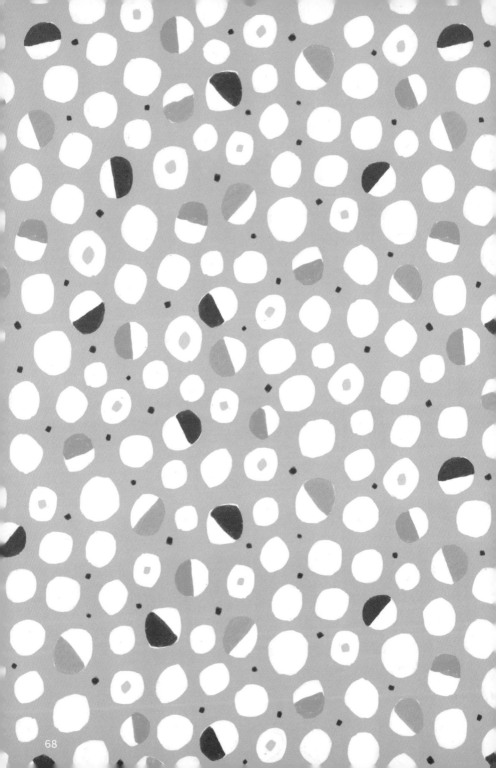

Let us make pregnancy
an occasion when we
appreciate our female bodies.

MERETE LEONHARDT-LUPA

My belly
is growing!

It's changed the way I...

_____

_____

_____

_____

_____

_____

_____

_____

_____

_____

_____

_____

_____

_____

_____

_____

_____

_____

As we get bigger, I like to think about...

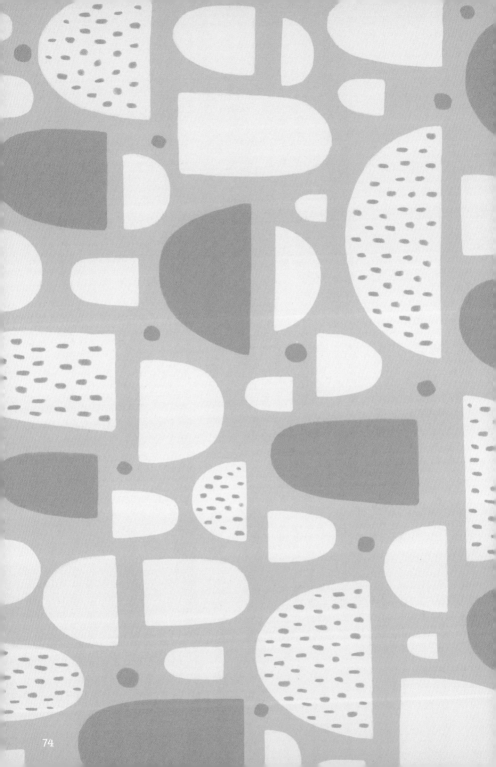

Pregnancy is a process
that invites you to
surrender to the unseen
force behind all life.

JUDY FORD

My birth plan:

I decided on this plan because...

_____

_____

_____

_____

_____

_____

_____

_____

_____

_____

_____

_____

_____

_____

_____

_____

_____

_____

_____

_____

_____

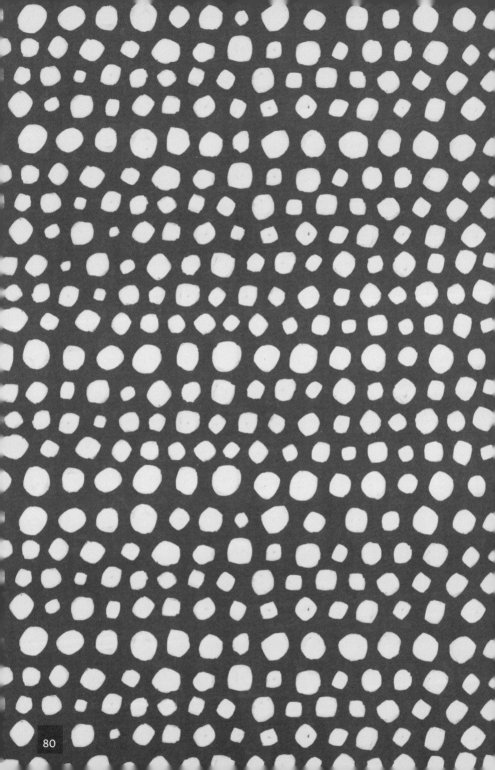

Being a mother is learning
about strengths you didn't know
you had... and dealing with
fears you didn't know existed.

LINDA WOOTEN

We're Growing!

WEEK:

You're the size of a:

These days I'm feeling:

_____
_____
_____
_____
_____
_____
_____
_____
_____
_____
_____
_____

Ways you've grown and developed recently:

_____
_____
_____
_____
_____
_____
_____
_____
_____
_____
_____
_____
_____

Right now, I'm most looking forward to:

I'm getting ready for you by:

NOTES

& THINGS TO REMEMBER

...what is done in

love is done well.

VINCENT VAN GOGH

How I'm preparing for the day you'll be born:

My hopes:

My fears:

Names

we're thinking of giving you:

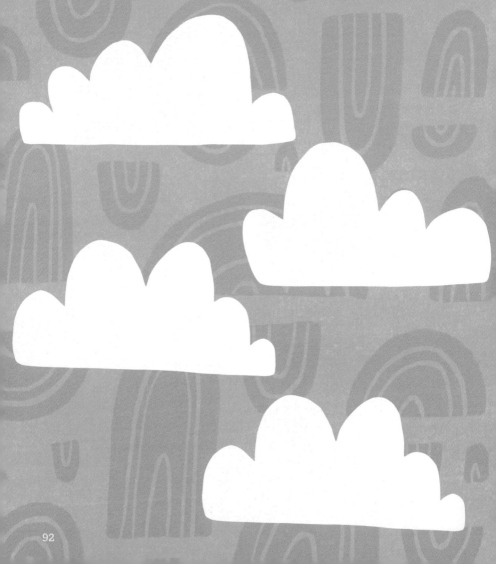

We like them because...

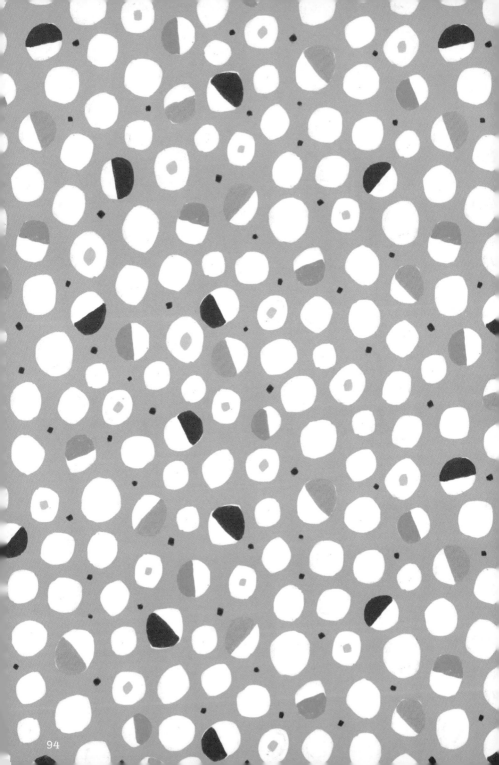

A baby fills a place

in your heart that you

never knew was empty.

ANONYMOUS

We're Growing!

WEEK:

You're the size of a:

These days I'm feeling:

Ways you've grown and developed recently:

Right now, I'm most looking forward to:

I'm getting ready for you by:

NOTES

& THINGS TO REMEMBER

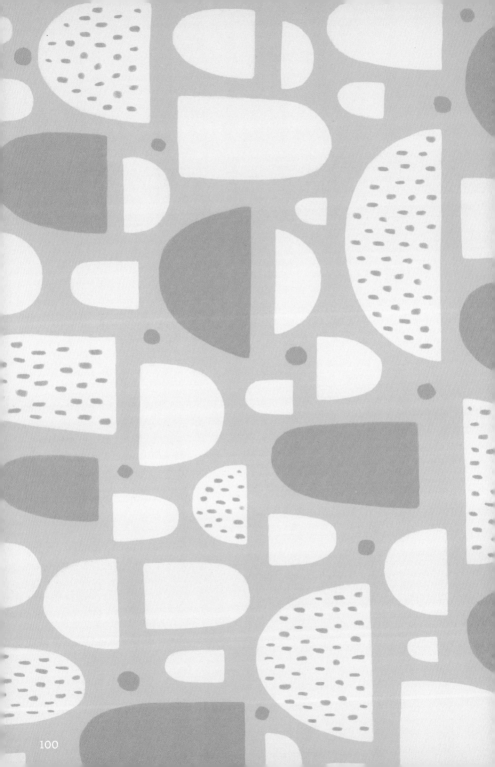

Whether your pregnancy
was meticulously planned,
medically coaxed, or happened by
surprise, one thing is certain—
your life will never be the same.

CATHERINE JONES

My favorite part about being pregnant:

My least favorite part about being pregnant:

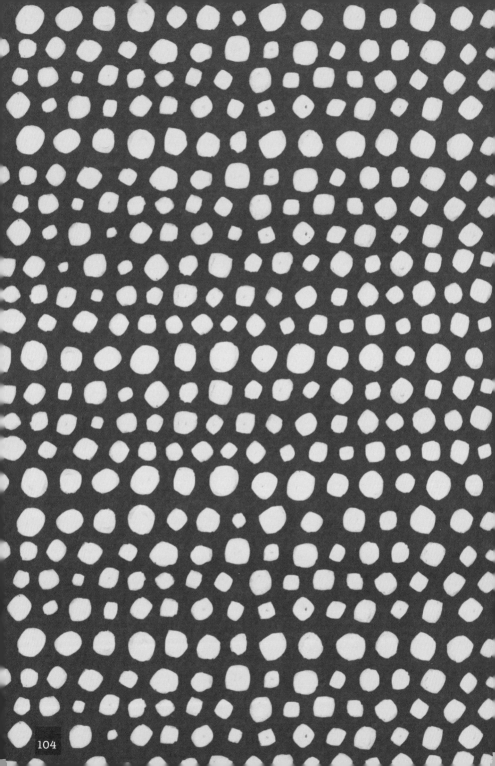

Loving a baby is a circular business, a kind of feedback loop. The more you give the more you get and the more you feel like giving.

PENELOPE LEACH

While you're still in my belly, we do special activities together.

From reading out loud to listening to music, some of
my favorite things to do with you and for you are...

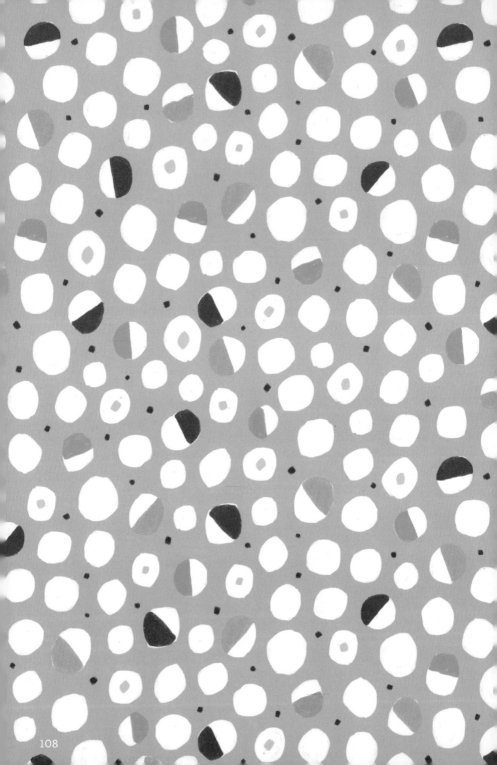

Life is always a rich
and steady time when
you are waiting for
something to happen...

E. B. WHITE

We're Growing!

WEEK:

You're the size of a:

These days I'm feeling:

Ways you've grown and developed recently:

Right now, I'm most looking forward to:

I'm getting ready for you by:

NOTES

& THINGS TO REMEMBER

How I feel when I talk to you:

_____
_____
_____
_____
_____
_____
_____
_____
_____
_____
_____
_____
_____
_____
_____
_____
_____
_____
_____
_____
_____
_____
_____
_____
_____

Things I like to say to you:

When you moved,
I felt squeezed with
a wild infatuation
and protectiveness.
We are one.

SUZANNE FINNAMORE

When you move, it feels like...

Hello to a new adventure.

ERNIE HARWELL

I have so many wonderful things ready for you.

Things we've purchased:

_____

_____

_____

_____

_____

_____

_____

_____

_____

_____

_____

_____

Thoughtful gifts we've received:

_____

_____

_____

_____

_____

_____

_____

_____

_____

_____

_____

_____

...life was made

for loving.

ELLA WHEELER WILCOX

We're Growing!

WEEK:

You're the size of a:

These days I'm feeling:

Ways you've grown and developed recently:

Right now, I'm most looking forward to:

I'm getting ready for you by:

NOTES

& THINGS TO REMEMBER

This is what your nursery looks like:

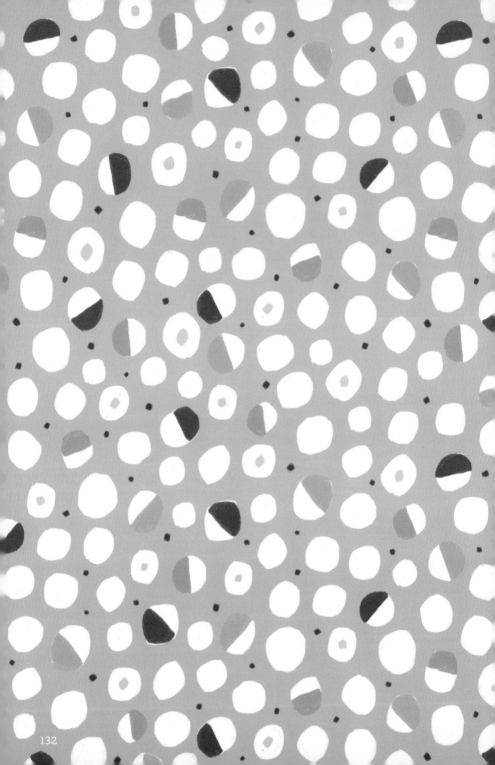

You are the poem I never knew how to write and this life is the story I have always wanted to tell.

TYLER KNOTT GREGSON

Soon, I'll hold you in my arms.

I can't wait to...

What I imagine it will be like when I see you
for the first time...

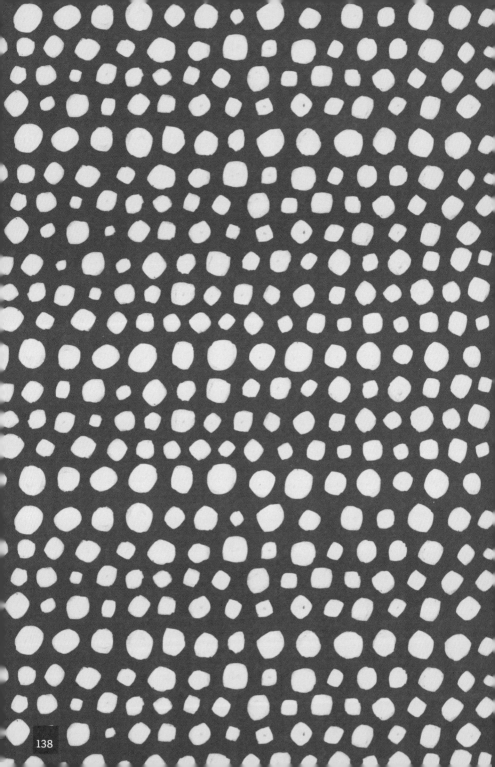

In giving birth to
our babies, we may
find that we give birth
to new possibilities
within ourselves.

MYLA & JON KABAT-ZINN

Oh! You're finally here!

We've chosen to name you:

No one understands
how someone so little can
so change their world—
until they hold their
baby in their arms.

PAM BROWN

When I first saw you...

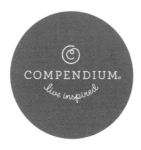

With special thanks to the entire Compendium family.

CREDITS:

Written and Compiled by: Amelia Riedler
Designed by: Justine Edge
Edited by: M.H. Clark and Ruth Austin

ISBN: 978-1-946873-87-3

1st printing. Printed in China with soy inks.